Masturbation Unveiled

Masturbation Unveiled

Solo to Sexual Health, Side Effects, and Breaking Free

Bruce P. Frye

Dedication

Dedicated to those embracing the journey of self-pleasure, self-discovery, and well-being, may this exploration of intimate health and liberation be a source of understanding and empowerment. Embrace self-pleasure mindfully for a healthier and happier you.

Contents

Dedication vi

Introduction 1

Chapter 1 The Fundamentals of Masturbation 7

- What is Masturbation? 7

- Significance of Masturbation 8

- Dispelling Myths about Masturbation..................9

Chapter 2 Masturbation Basics 13

- Understanding the Complexities of Genital Anatomy..13

- How to Explore and Experiment with Your Body 15

Chapter 3 Masturbation and Sexual Health 19

- The Connection Between Masturbation and Sexual Well-being...19

- Exploring How Masturbation Enhances Sexual Function and Performance Masturbation. 20

- Masturbation and sexual dysfunction / brokenness 23

- How to Cope with Sexual Dysfunction (Sexual Brokenness) Induced by Masturbating...............27

- Signs of sexual dysfunction / Brokenness..........28

- How to Handle Masturbation-Induced Sexual Dysfunction 30

Chapter 4 Benefits of Masturbation................................. 33

- Health Benefit 33

- Distance Relationship..36

Chapter 5 Masturbation and Relationships......................39

- How Masturbation can Improve Your Sex Life with Your Partner..39

- Understanding Your Partner's Masturbation Habits 41

- Addressing Envy and Insecurity Associated with Masturbation in Relationships..........................43

- Mutual Masturbation and Its Advantages 45

Chapter 6: Masturbation and Gender...............................47

- Masturbation and Orientation..........................47

- Orientation Dysphoria and Masturbation..........48

Chapter 7: Masturbation and Culture.............................51

- Masturbation in Various Societies 51

- Masturbation and religion 52

- General Considerations 54

- Masturbation and Public Shame.......................55

Chapter 8: How to Stop Masturbation 59

- Identifying Triggers..59

Conclusion 63

Say no to porn...65

Try Something else 65

Seek expert guidance. 66

Spend a ton of time mingling 66

Regular actual work...67

POEM 69

- Health Benefit of Masturbation...........................69
Health Challenge of Excessive Masturbation 72
Why to Stop Excessive Masturbation 73

Introduction

Let's talk about a topic that has often been shrouded in stigma and taboo but is, in fact, a natural and healthy aspect of human sexuality—masturbation. A simple act that involves the self-stimulation of one's own genital organs for pleasure, masturbation has been a subject of curiosity, myths, and misconceptions throughout history.

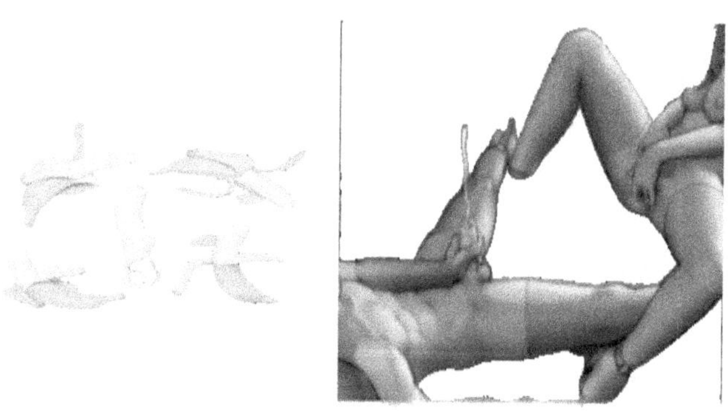

Historical Perspectives

In the past, masturbation was clouded with superstitions and strict taboos, condemned by religious and moral teachings.

The Old Testament story of Onan portrayed it as a sinful act, and many premodern societies frowned upon it during the maturity phase of human development. However, societal attitudes have evolved over time, and the stigma surrounding masturbation has gradually diminished.

Changing Perceptions

In the mid-20th century, researchers like Alfred Kinsey challenged prevailing notions, estimating that a significant percentage of the population, around 92% of American males and 70-80% of females, engaged in masturbation. Today, attitudes are shifting, and scholars of sexual behavior recognize its potential benefits—considering it a healthy, pleasurable, and stress-relieving activity.

The Modern Perspective

This book delves into the exploration of masturbation from a contemporary standpoint. Written with a focus on accurate information, research, and the de-stigmatization of this natural sexual expression, it aims to provide you with insights, tools, and techniques to understand and embrace your own sexuality. Despite the progress we've made, there is still lingering shame associated with masturbation, and this book seeks to dispel myths and foster a positive view of self-pleasure.

Breaking Barriers

Whether influenced by religious beliefs, societal norms, or personal reservations, the goal is to encourage a healthy sexual life by recognizing masturbation as a legitimate and personal choice. This book aims to empower you with knowledge and resources, reinforcing the idea that masturbation is a safe and natural part of human sexuality.

Conclusion

Masturbation, far from being a clandestine or taboo subject, is presented here as a natural and normal form of sexual expression. It is a private, individual activity that transcends gender and sexual orientation, offering a range of physical and psychological benefits.

As you embark on this exploration of self-pleasure, remember that everyone has their own comfort levels, and the key is to approach it safely, respectfully, and consensually.

Chapter 1 The Fundamentals of Masturbation

What is Masturbation?

Masturbation is the act of stimulating one's own genitalia for sexual gratification, a natural and common human behavior that can be performed individually or with a partner.

It involves various methods, such as using hands, sex toys, or other items, providing a healthy and safe means of achieving orgasm, releasing sexual tension, and exploring one's sexuality.

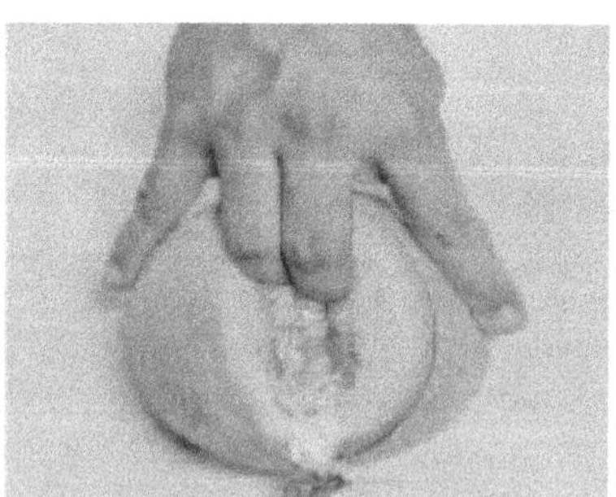

Masturbation A Personal Choice

While masturbation is widely accepted, it remains a personal choice, and some individuals may choose not to engage in this form of self-stimulation. Preferences regarding sexual practices can vary, and it's essential to respect individual choices.

Significance of Masturbation

Masturbation plays a crucial role in the development of a healthy sexuality. It serves as a natural and routine way to understand one's body, experience pleasure, and achieve climax.

Whether using hands, fingers, sex toys, or other means, masturbation enables individuals to explore physical preferences, fostering sexual satisfaction and boosting self-confidence.

Benefits of Masturbation

Engaging in masturbation has significant positive effects on both physical and mental well-being. By triggering the release of feel-good chemicals like endorphins and oxytocin, it helps alleviate stress.

Masturbation promotes relaxation, reduces tension, and can contribute to improved sleep quality. Additionally, it enhances muscle tone and facilitates blood flow to the genital area, potentially improving sexual performance.

Dispelling Myths about Masturbation

Masturbation has been subject to various myths and misconceptions, leading to feelings of guilt, shame, and confusion. Addressing these myths is crucial for fostering a healthy understanding of human sexuality.

Myth 1 Masturbation is Only for Loners

Contrary to the misconception that masturbation is exclusive to lonely or sexually deprived individuals, it is a normal practice regardless of relationship status. Many people in content and happy relationships still choose to masturbate as a natural aspect of self-exploration.

Myth 2 Masturbation Harms Physical or Mental Health

There is no evidence supporting the notion that masturbation harms physical or mental health. On the contrary, it offers numerous health benefits, including stress reduction, mood enhancement, and improved sleep. It also aids in self-awareness of one's body and sexual preferences, contributing positively to relationships and sexual health.

Myth 3 Only Men Masturbate

Dispelling the myth that masturbation is solely a male activity is crucial. Women also engage in masturbation, finding it to be a positive and enjoyable aspect of their sexual lives. Many women express that masturbation provides more gratifying orgasms than actual sexual activity.

Myth 4 Masturbation Indicates Sexual Addiction

While some individuals may develop a masturbation addiction, it is inaccurate to assume that everyone who masturbates has such an issue. Most people engage in masturbation as a regular and healthy practice without experiencing negative consequences associated with addiction, such as a loss of control.

In conclusion, dispelling myths surrounding masturbation is essential, as it is a natural and healthy element of human sexuality. Providing accurate information fosters comfort and security in individuals exploring their bodies and sexual desires.

Chapter 2 Masturbation Basics

Understanding the Complexities of Genital Anatomy

Genitalia, the external sex organs responsible for both reproduction and sexual pleasure, play a vital role in sexual health and satisfaction. Let's delve into the detailed anatomy of both male and female genitalia.

Men's Genitalia

The male genitalia comprise the penis and scrotum. The penis, with its root, shaft, and glans, is a cylindrical organ. The root anchors to the pubic bone, and the urethra, responsible for urine and semen elimination, runs through the shaft.

The glans, highly sensitive to touch, crowns the penis. The testes, housed in the scrotum, produce testosterone and sperm, and the scrotum regulates their temperature for optimal functioning.

Women's Genitalia

Female genitalia include the vulva, clitoris, vagina, cervix, and uterus. The vulva consists of the labia majora, labia minora, clitoris, and vaginal entrance. The labia majora are external lips, while the labia minora are inner lips.

The clitoris, a sensitive organ at the vulva's apex, contributes to sexual pleasure. The vagina, a muscular canal, connects the vulva and cervix. The cervix is the lower part of the uterus, and the uterus, crucial for menstruation and pregnancy, houses the fallopian tubes connecting to the ovaries, the female reproductive glands.

Navigating Sexual Wellness in Elders

For elders, maintaining sexual wellness is an integral part of overall well-being. Understanding the changes in genital anatomy that come with age is crucial. Both men and women may experience shifts in hormone levels, affecting sexual desire and function. Open communication with healthcare providers about sexual health concerns is vital for seniors to navigate this aspect of their well-being.

Both male and female genitalia are highly sensitive and contribute to sexual pleasure. Understanding this intricate anatomy can enhance sexual health and enjoyment. It's crucial to recognize that genitals come in diverse sizes and shapes, and there is no singular "correct" or "normal" appearance.

How to Explore and Experiment with Your Body

Create a Comfortable Setting

Set the mood with aromatic candles, soothing music, and dim lighting for a pleasurable masturbation experience.

Experiment with Methods

Try various techniques like massaging, caressing, tapping, or incorporating sex toys. Adjust the pace and pressure to find what works for you.

Explore Erogenous Zones

Discover and stimulate erogenous zones, such as the clitoris, penis, nipples, anus, and neck, which vary from person to person.

Use Lubrication

Enhance your sexual encounter with suitable lubrication that works well with your body and any sex gadgets you may use.

Self-Discovery

Pay attention to your body's reactions and explore your fantasies and desires during masturbation.

Practice Safe Sex

If using sex toys, ensure proper cleaning before and after each use. Use condoms when sharing toys or if concerns about STDs arise.

Remember, masturbation is a natural and common method to explore your body and sexuality, offering positive psychological and physical effects, such as stress reduction and relaxation. For seniors, incorporating sexual wellness into their overall health is part of aging gracefully.

Chapter 3 Masturbation and Sexual Health

The Connection Between Masturbation and Sexual Well-being

Masturbation is a common and healthy sexual behavior that plays a significant role in enhancing an individual's sexual life.

It involves the physical stimulation of one's own private parts and serves as a way for individuals to understand their bodies better, facilitating more effective communication of preferences and desires in sexual interactions with others.

This practice can help release sexual tension and alleviate stress, potentially benefiting those dealing with issues like erectile dysfunction or premature ejaculation.

However, it is crucial to acknowledge that excessive masturbation may have adverse effects such as desensitization, decreased libido, and challenges in achieving orgasm during sexual activity with a partner.

Exploring How Masturbation Enhances Sexual Function and Performance Masturbation.

often subjected to misconceptions, is, in fact, a natural and beneficial form of sexual expression that can contribute to improved sexual function and performance. Let's delve into how engaging in this practice can enhance these aspects.

Boosting Sexual Arousal and Desire

Masturbation stimulates erogenous zones, leading to increased sexual arousal and desire. Regular practice can also enhance libido by reducing stress and tension, common hindrances to sexual desire.

Enhancing Sexual Confidence and Awareness

By allowing individuals to explore their own bodies, masturbation promotes sexual confidence and self-awareness. This can be particularly beneficial for those seeking to build sexual confidence or express preferences to their partners.

Improving Control Over Sexual Responses

Masturbation serves as a form of sexual practice, enabling individuals to learn how to manage their sexual responses, including arousal levels, timing of orgasm, and ejaculation. This can be valuable for those dealing with premature ejaculation or aiming to enhance sexual endurance.

Elevating the Quality of Orgasm

Understanding what sensations and stimuli lead to a satisfying climax is an insight gained through masturbation. This knowledge can be applied to sexual activities with a partner, increasing the likelihood of achieving a more fulfilling orgasm.

Promoting Sexual Health

Regular masturbation can enhance blood flow to the genitals, potentially improving sexual performance and reducing the risk of erectile dysfunction. It may also contribute to prostate health by flushing potentially harmful toxins from the prostate gland.

In conclusion, masturbation can be a valuable component of a person's sexual life, offering benefits such as stress relief, improved sexual confidence, and better control over sexual responses.

However, like any sexual activity, moderation and respect for individual and partner preferences should be maintained for a healthy and satisfying sexual experience.

Masturbation contributes to improved sexual capability and performance by alleviating sexual anxiety and stress. Serving as a form of stress release, masturbation aids individuals in reducing levels of sexual uneasiness and tension, offering particular benefits for those grappling with sexual anxiety or dysfunction induced by stress.

Furthermore, masturbation enhances sexual capability and performance by fostering a positive attitude toward sex. It helps individuals become more comfortable with their own sexuality, leading to an overall healthier perspective on sex. This can be especially beneficial for those who have experienced sexual trauma or had negative sexual encounters in the past.

In summary, masturbation is a natural and healthy method of sexual expression that enhances sexual capability and performance in various ways.

It boosts sexual arousal and desire, improves sexual confidence and awareness, aids in controlling sexual responses, enhances the quality of orgasms, improves sexual health, reduces sexual anxiety and stress, and nurtures a positive attitude toward sex.

As a result, individuals are encouraged to explore their own bodies through masturbation to enhance their sexual capability and performance.

Masturbation and sexual dysfunction / brokenness

Masturbation and sexual dysfunction are often used interchangeably, assuming that one leads to the other. Masturbation involves self-stimulation of one's genitals for sexual pleasure or climax, while sexual dysfunction refers to the inability to achieve or sustain an erection, orgasm, or sexual desire.

Let's explore the relationship between masturbation and sexual dysfunction, exploring the causes, effects, and potential treatments.

Masturbation, a practice spanning generations, is considered normal and healthy in many cultures. However, some religious and social groups view it as immoral or indecent.

Research indicates that masturbation offers various health benefits, including stress relief, improved sleep, and heightened sexual pleasure. It can also aid individuals in exploring their bodies, fostering a deeper awareness of their sexual needs and preferences.

On the other hand, sexual dysfunction encompasses various issues that can arise during sexual engagement, such as difficulty achieving or maintaining an erection, premature or delayed ejaculation, and poor sexual desire.

Causes include medical conditions like diabetes or heart disease, psychological issues like anxiety or depression, certain medications, and a lack of sexual experience or education leading to discomfort during sexual engagement.

The relationship between masturbation and sexual dysfunction is complex and varied. Some studies suggest that frequent masturbation may contribute to sexual dysfunction, while others argue that it can help prevent it.

The frequency and intensity of masturbation play crucial roles in this interaction.

Studies propose that regular and intense masturbation might lead to nerve desensitization in the genital area, making it challenging to achieve or maintain an erection during sexual activity.

This condition, known as "sexual fatigue," can affect individuals of all genders and may cause a decline in sexual desire and overall satisfaction. However, it's crucial to note that sexual fatigue is a rare condition generally observed in those engaging in excessively frequent or intense masturbation.

Conversely, several studies demonstrate that masturbation can contribute to preventing sexual dysfunction. It can help individuals feel more comfortable with their bodies and sexual desires, leading to enhanced sexual confidence and overall improvement in sexual capability.

Additionally, regular masturbation can aid in maintaining optimal sexual function by improving blood flow to the genital region and preventing sexual dysfunction caused by physical illnesses like diabetes or heart disease.

Age can significantly impact the relationship between masturbation and sexual dysfunction. As individuals age, their sexual capability typically decreases, resulting in a decline in sexual desire, difficulties in achieving or maintaining an erection, and other forms of sexual dysfunction.

Masturbation can assist older individuals in maintaining healthy sexual function by increasing blood flow to the genital area and keeping the nerves in that area strong and open.

It's crucial to emphasize that masturbation is not a cure for sexual dysfunction. If an individual is experiencing sexual dysfunction, consulting with a healthcare provider is essential to identify the underlying cause and devise an effective treatment strategy.

Moreover, excessive masturbation may signal an underlying mental health issue, such as anxiety or depression, which can also contribute to sexual dysfunction.

In conclusion, the relationship between masturbation and sexual dysfunction is nuanced and diverse. While frequent and intense masturbation may lead to sexual fatigue and potentially contribute to sexual dysfunction, regular masturbation can offer benefits to individuals, especially when practiced in moderation.

How to Cope with Sexual Dysfunction (Sexual Brokenness) Induced by Masturbating

Sexual dysfunction is a prevalent issue affecting individuals of all genders and is caused by a range of factors, encompassing mental, physiological, and social challenges. Masturbation is identified as one of the contributors to sexual dysfunction, with its impact being more common in men than in women. Coping with masturbation-related sexual dysfunction can be challenging, but various methods exist to address this issue.

Despite its potential benefits, excessive masturbation can lead to sexual dysfunction, including erectile dysfunction, premature ejaculation, and delayed ejaculation. Moreover, masturbation can contribute to mental health problems such as anxiety, depression, and diminished self-esteem, further exacerbating issues related to sexual health.

Signs of sexual dysfunction / Brokenness

1. Difficulty acquiring or maintaining an erection

This sign, often associated with erectile dysfunction, refers to the inability to achieve or sustain an erection sufficient for sexual activity. It can result from various factors such as age, underlying health conditions, psychological issues, or a combination of these.

2. Excessive ejaculation or difficulty ejaculating

This sign indicates irregularities in the ejaculation process. It can manifest as either premature ejaculation (releasing too quickly) or difficulty ejaculating, which may be linked to psychological factors, hormonal imbalances, or certain medications.

3. Delayed ejaculation causing difficulty in releasing

Delayed ejaculation involves a prolonged time to reach orgasm or difficulty in ejaculating despite sufficient sexual stimulation. Psychological factors, medications, or neurological issues could contribute to this condition.

4. Reduced sexual desire or libido

A decrease in sexual desire or libido means experiencing a diminished interest in sexual activities. This can be influenced by factors such as hormonal changes, stress, relationship issues, or underlying health conditions.

5. Pain or discomfort during sexual activity

Pain or discomfort during sexual activity may result from various causes, including infections, anatomical issues, psychological factors, or underlying health conditions. It's crucial to address this symptom promptly to identify and treat the root cause.

Understanding these signs is essential for individuals experiencing sexual dysfunction or brokenness, as they can serve as indicators prompting further investigation into potential causes and appropriate treatment options. Consulting with a healthcare professional is crucial to assess individual cases and determine the most effective course of action.

How to Handle Masturbation-Induced Sexual Dysfunction

1. Consult with a Clinical Professional

Seeking advice from a healthcare professional is crucial for understanding and addressing the root cause of masturbation-induced sexual dysfunction. A doctor or therapist can provide guidance and recommend appropriate treatment options, possibly referring the individual to a specialist if needed.

2. Make Lifestyle Changes

Adopting healthier lifestyle habits can positively impact sexual function. Regular exercise, a nutritious diet, avoiding smoking, limiting alcohol intake, ensuring sufficient sleep, managing stress, and maintaining a healthy weight can contribute to overall well-being and, in turn, influence sexual function.

3. Practice Mindfulness Techniques

Mindfulness practices such as meditation, yoga, and deep breathing can help reduce stress and anxiety, contributing to improved sexual function. These techniques enhance self-awareness, helping individuals recognize and manage any issues they may be facing.

4. Consider Treatment

Therapy, especially Cognitive-Behavioral Therapy (CBT), can be beneficial in identifying and modifying negative thought patterns linked to sexual dysfunction. Couples counseling may also be effective in addressing relationship-related stressors impacting sexual function.

5. Explore Medication Options

Medications like sildenafil (Viagra), tadalafil (Cialis), and vardenafil (Levitra) can enhance erectile function by increasing blood flow to the penis. However, it is essential to consult with a healthcare professional before taking any medication for sexual dysfunction, as they may have side effects and interactions with other drugs.

6. Consider Alternative Treatments

Alternative treatments such as acupuncture, herbal supplements, and massage therapies may assist some individuals in improving sexual function. However, it is crucial to consult with a healthcare professional before trying any alternative treatments to ensure safety and compatibility with other medications.

7. Experiment with Various Sexual Strategies

Exploring alternative sexual practices like mutual masturbation, oral sex, and manual stimulation can provide sexual satisfaction without relying on penetration. This can help alleviate performance anxiety and enhance overall sexual function.

Chapter 4 Benefits of Masturbation

Health Benefit

1. Stress Reduction

Masturbation triggers the release of endorphins, natural substances that reduce tension and promote relaxation. It can contribute to stress relief, helping individuals to relax and potentially improve sleep quality.

2. Better Sexual Functionality

Regular and healthy masturbation aids individuals in understanding their bodies and sexual responses, leading to more satisfying sexual experiences. It can also enhance sexual endurance and reduce the risk of sexual dysfunctions like premature ejaculation and erectile dysfunction.

3. Pain Relief

Masturbation can alleviate pain, including menstrual discomfort, headaches, and other types of pain. The release of endorphins during masturbation has analgesic properties similar to natural painkillers.

4. Improved Immune Function

Masturbation can support the immune system by increasing white blood cell production. White blood cells play a crucial role in fighting infections and diseases, contributing to overall immune function.

5. Lower Prostate Cancer Risk

Regular masturbation in men has been linked to a reduced occurrence of prostate cancer. Those who masturbate regularly have a lower risk of developing prostate cancer compared to those who do not.

6. Enhanced Mood

Masturbation can enhance mood and alleviate symptoms of depression and anxiety. The release of endorphins during masturbation contributes to an improved mood, increased feelings of pleasure, and overall well-being.

7. Enhanced Sexual Confidence

Regular masturbation helps individuals become more familiar with their bodies and sexual responses, leading to increased sexual confidence in various settings.

8. Improved Heart Health

By reducing stress and promoting relaxation, masturbation has been associated with improved heart health. It has been linked to a decreased risk of cardiovascular disease and stroke.

9. Enhanced Mental Performance

Increased blood flow to the brain during masturbation can improve mental performance. The release of endorphins contributes to enhanced mental clarity and cognitive function.

10. Preserving Intimacy in Distant Relationships

Masturbation can help maintain intimacy in long-distance relationships by allowing partners to experience sexual pleasure and intimacy even when physically apart.

In summary, masturbation is described as a healthy and natural sexual practice with numerous benefits, including stress relief, enhanced sexual functionality, pain relief, improved immune function, reduced risk of prostate cancer, mood enhancement, increased sexual confidence, improved heart health, enhanced mental performance, and preserving intimacy in distant relationships. The overall portrayal suggests that masturbation is a safe and healthy way to explore one's sexuality while promoting overall health and well-being.

Distance Relationship

It assists couples with communicating their sexual requirements and inclinations.

Masturbation permits accomplices to investigate their bodies and get more familiar with what they view as fulfilling. They can help with laying out a superior information on one another's sexual necessities and inclinations by imparting this data to their accomplice.

It guides in the support of sexual closeness.

Masturbation can help with the support of sexual closeness in a remote relationship. Accomplices can keep up with sexual closeness with each other even while they are separated by taking part in independent sexual action.

It can work on sexual correspondence.

Masturbation between couples can be a sort of sexual correspondence. Accomplices can foster a superior information on one another's sexual requirements and inclinations by trading insights concerning their independent sexual experiences, which can prompt more wonderful sexual encounters when they are together face to face.

It can help with the decrease of sexual disappointment.
Sexual disappointment is an ordinary issue in far-removed relationships. At the point when darlings can't be together

face to face, masturbation can assist them with delivering sexual pressure and disappointment.

Masturbation can be a kind of sexual trial and error. Masturbation can be a method for couples to evaluate new sexual procedures or dreams. They can keep on investigating their sexual advantages and needs even while they are isolated by talking about these encounters.

In general, masturbation can assist accomplices with keeping closeness in lengthy separation connections by permitting them to communicate their sexual longings and inclinations, keep up with sexual closeness, work on sexual correspondence, diminish sexual disappointment, and trial physically.

Chapter 5 Masturbation and Relationships

How Masturbation can Improve Your Sex Life with Your Partner

Masturbation is a completely normal and healthy form of sexual expression that can prove beneficial to individuals and their sexual experiences with their partners in various ways. Masturbation can enhance your sexual life with your life partner in the following ways

1. Increased Awareness and Confidence

Explanation Masturbation helps individuals explore their bodies, needs, and preferences in a non-judgmental and comfortable environment, leading to better awareness and confidence. This, in turn, can result in more satisfying sexual experiences with a partner.

2. Improved Sexual Proficiency

Explanation Regular masturbation can help individuals become more comfortable with their sexual responses, contributing to better sexual proficiency during partnered sex. This may include increased desire, improved ejaculation control, and a greater ability to achieve climax.

3. Increased Sexual Pleasure

Explanation Masturbation enables individuals to discover new erogenous zones or stimulation techniques they might not have found otherwise. As individuals express their desires to their partners, this can lead to increased sexual satisfaction during partnered sex.

4. Reduced Performance Anxiety

Explanation Masturbation aids in reducing performance anxiety by allowing individuals to experiment with new techniques and gain confidence in their sexual abilities without the pressure of a partner. This can result in a more relaxed and enjoyable sexual experience with a partner.

5. Improved Communication

Explanation Masturbation helps individuals feel more comfortable discussing their sexual needs and preferences with their partner, fostering a more open and enjoyable conversation during partnered sex.

In summary, masturbation can be a useful approach for increasing sexual experiences with a partner. Individuals may have more meaningful and rewarding sexual experiences with their partners through improved awareness, sexual proficiency, pleasure, and communication.

Understanding Your Partner's Masturbation Habits

Masturbation is a natural and healthy aspect of human sexuality, and many individuals engage in it regardless of their relationship circumstances. When in a romantic relationship, it's crucial to understand and respect each other's sexual needs and preferences, including masturbation practices.

Understanding your partner's masturbation habits could assist in building a better and more intimate connection. It can help you comprehend their sexual desires and preferences, leading to a more significant and satisfying sexual life for both of you.

Knowing what your partner enjoys for solo play allows you to incorporate these preferences into your sexual activities together, potentially enhancing your sexual experiences.

Furthermore, sharing your masturbation practices with your partner could help build trust and communication in your relationship. It can facilitate a more open dialogue about sex, leading to better sexual communication overall. Knowing that you and your partner are openly discussing masturbation can also help reduce any feelings of shame or guilt associated with the act.

In conclusion, understanding your partner's masturbation habit is a fundamental aspect of a healthy and successful sexual relationship. It can support the development of trust, communication, and intimacy, resulting in a more enjoyable sexual life for both you and your partner.

Addressing Envy and Insecurity Associated with Masturbation in Relationships

Masturbation-related envy and insecurity in relationships can be challenging to address, but they are essential for maintaining a healthy and rewarding relationship. Here are various ways to approach the issue

1. Communication is Essential

Explanation The first step is to have an open dialogue about how you are feeling with your partner. It is crucial to approach the conversation with empathy and compassion rather than blaming or accusing. Instead of attacking your partner, focus on communicating how you feel and why you have that impression.

2. Determine the Source of the Issue

Explanation Identifying the source of your jealousy and insecurity is crucial. Is it because you lack trust in your partner? Do you feel somewhat insecure about your sexual preferences and needs? Understanding the source of the issue can allow you and your partner to genuinely address it.

3. Examine Your Views

Explanation Your jealousy and insecurity are likely the results of incorrect beliefs or societal norms. Reflect on these views and where they originated. Masturbation is a common and healthy form of sexual expression that does not necessarily reflect the strength of your relationship.

4. Establish Limits

Explanation If certain aspects of your partner's masturbation habits make you uncomfortable, setting boundaries is essential. Collaborate to determine what is and isn't acceptable in your relationship.

5. Seek Professional Help

Explanation If your jealousy and insecurity are causing significant distress and negatively impacting your relationship, it could be beneficial to seek professional help from a therapist or counselor who can provide guidance and support.

In conclusion, addressing jealousy and insecurity in relationships requires a willingness to have an open conversation, a commitment to understanding and addressing the root of the problem, and a readiness to collaborate to establish boundaries and find a solution that works for both partners.

Mutual Masturbation and Its Advantages

Mutual masturbation is a form of sexual expression in which two individuals engage in self-pleasure in the presence of each other. It's a playful method to explore sexual desires while enhancing intimacy between lovers.

One of the benefits of mutual masturbation is that it allows couples to openly share their sexual preferences and desires. This can help build trust and communication in the relationship, leading to a happier sexual life.

Mutual masturbation also helps couples explore their bodies and learn about their pleasure in a safe, non-judgmental setting, resulting in improved awareness and confidence, contributing to overall better sexual experiences.

Mutual masturbation enjoys another benefit in that it enables partners to engage in sexual activity without the risk of pregnancy or sexually transmitted diseases (STDs). This is especially crucial for couples who are not ready or interested in having sexual intercourse.

Overall, mutual masturbation is a unique and beneficial method for couples to explore their sexuality and deepen their relationship connection.

Chapter 6: Masturbation and Gender

Masturbation and Orientation

Masturbation is a natural and normal aspect of human sexuality that is not inherently associated with a specific orientation. Individuals of both genders engage in masturbation for various reasons, including stress reduction, body exploration, and sexual satisfaction.

However, societal and cultural perspectives about masturbation vary depending on orientation. Historically, female masturbation has been stigmatized and prohibited, with women often facing embarrassment or punishment for engaging in self-pleasure.

This is partly due to outdated notions about women's sexual desires and the traditional assumption that women are sexually passive.

On the other hand, male masturbation has often been permitted and even encouraged, with male sexuality frequently celebrated and considered a natural aspect of masculinity. However, this may lead to harmful biases and put pressure on men to perform sexually at all times.

It is crucial to recognize that everyone's experiences with masturbation and orientation are unique, and there is no "right" or "wrong" way to feel or express one's sexuality. Emphasizing personal pleasure and consent is critical, as is creating a culture that honors and respects all forms of sexual expression, regardless of orientation.

Orientation Dysphoria and Masturbation

Orientation dysphoria is a condition where an individual feel distressed or uncomfortable due to a misalignment between their gender identity and the sex assigned to them at birth. Masturbation can be a challenging topic for those with orientation dysphoria, as it may trigger feelings of discomfort about their body and gender identity.

For instance, a transgender person experiencing dysphoria about their genitalia may feel uneasy or upset while masturbating. They might be uncomfortable with the physical sensations or mental images associated with their assigned gender.

It is important to note, however, that not all transgender individuals experience masturbation-related dysphoria. Some may find that it alleviates dysphoria by allowing them to explore their bodies and sexuality in an authentic and affirming manner.

If an individual with orientation dysphoria is experiencing pain or distress due to masturbation, they should seek support from a mental health professional knowledgeable about gender identity concerns.

This may involve exploring ways to reduce discomfort while masturbating or finding alternative forms of sexual expression that are more comfortable and affirming.

Ultimately, individuals with orientation dysphoria should prioritize their own physical and personal well-being and find ways to express their sexuality in manners that feel authentic and fulfilling to them.

Chapter 7: Masturbation and Culture

Masturbation in Various Societies

Masturbation is perceived differently across various cultures and religions, ranging from acceptance to judgment.

Natural and Healthy

In some cultures, masturbation is considered a natural and safe method to explore one's sexuality and release sexual tension. This perspective is prevalent in many secular Western countries.

Considered Sinful

In contrast, certain fundamentalist Christian and Muslim groups view masturbation as a form of immoral behavior and a violation of religious norms. In these societies, masturbation might be seen as extramarital perversion and a breach of religious regulations.

Not Discussed or Acknowledged

In some cultures, masturbation is not openly discussed and may be considered a private matter. It might be seen as a taboo topic that is not addressed publicly.

Masturbation and religion

Views on masturbation can vary within religious communities, and perspectives may differ among individuals within the same faith. It's important to note that interpretations and beliefs can evolve over time, and there may be diversity of thought within religious traditions. Here is a general overview:

Christianity

Catholicism

The Catholic Church historically viewed masturbation as a sinful act, considering it a violation of natural law and the purpose of sexual activity. The Catechism of the Catholic Church discourages masturbation, emphasizing the importance of sexual acts within marriage for procreation.

Protestant Denominations

Views on masturbation can vary among Protestant denominations. Some conservative branches might consider it a sin, while more liberal denominations may be more permissive, recognizing the role of individual conscience.

Islam

Traditional Islamic views on masturbation vary. While some scholars consider it impermissible, others suggest that it might be allowed in certain circumstances, such as to avoid adultery or for health reasons. The primary focus is often on maintaining chastity outside of marriage.

Hinduism

Hinduism encompasses diverse beliefs and practices, leading to varied perspectives on masturbation. Some Hindu traditions emphasize self-discipline and control over desires, potentially viewing masturbation negatively. Others may be more permissive, recognizing individual autonomy.

General Considerations

Evolution of Views

It's essential to recognize that religious views on masturbation can evolve, and interpretations may differ among believers and religious leaders. Some contemporary religious thinkers adopt more nuanced perspectives, acknowledging the complexities of human sexuality.

Individual Interpretation

The personal views of believers within each religion can differ widely. Some individuals may align closely with traditional teachings, while others may adopt more progressive or liberal stances, interpreting religious guidance in light of contemporary understanding.

Given the diversity of beliefs within religious communities, individuals seeking guidance on this matter are encouraged to consult with religious leaders, scholars, or authorities within their specific faith tradition for more tailored and accurate information.

Masturbation and Public Shame

Masturbation, the act of self-stimulation to achieve sexual pleasure and possibly orgasm, is a normal and frequent human behavior that is neither harmful nor dangerous. Despite its simplicity, many individuals experience shame or guilt regarding masturbation, often influenced by societal or cultural influences that perceive sexuality as taboo or sinful.

Shame is a complex emotion that can have severe implications for one's mental and personal well-being. It may lead individuals to feel guilty or embarrassed about their sexuality, resulting in low self-esteem and, in some cases, psychological distress related to masturbation.

Potential connections between shame and masturbation include

Social Conditioning

Society frequently portrays masturbation as incorrect, dirty, or shameful, especially for women. Messages from religious beliefs, cultural practices, or family values can contribute to these perceptions.

Lack of Education

Incomplete sex education, which excludes information about masturbation, can lead to misunderstandings or misinformation, exacerbating feelings of shame.

Sexual Trauma or Abuse

For some individuals, past sexual abuse or trauma can lead to feelings of shame about their sexuality, including masturbation. People may internalize their own challenging beliefs or attitudes toward masturbation, fostering feelings of shame or guilt.

Overcoming shame related to masturbation can involve recognizing and questioning the social and cultural messages that contribute to these negative emotions. Self-education about the benefits and safety of masturbation, along with self-reflection and self-compassion, can be beneficial.

Therapy or counseling can also address underlying psychological issues associated with shame and sexuality. Overcoming guilt about masturbation can ultimately lead to a happier and more fulfilling sexual life.

Chapter 8: How to Stop Masturbation

Identifying Triggers

Understanding Personal Triggers

Identify situations or factors that lead to the desire to masturbate. This could include boredom, stress, exposure to specific content, or other personal circumstances.

Stressful situations at work triggering the need for stress relief through masturbation.

Addressing Triggers

1. Avoidance or Control: Once triggers are identified, take measures to avoid or control them.

Developing stress-management techniques or finding alternative ways to cope with boredom.

2. Individual Variations: Acknowledge that people's preferences and triggers may change over time or fluctuate based on mood and circumstances.

A change in relationship status influencing one's sexual desires.

Overcoming Masturbation

1. Establishing Health-Promoting Habits: Develop positive routines that engage your time and energy in activities such as exercise, meditation, reading, or spending time with loved ones.

Engaging in regular physical activity to channel energy positively.

2. Avoiding Pornographic Material: If pornography is a trigger, limit exposure as much as possible. This may involve reducing internet time, avoiding specific websites, or installing software to block sexual content.

Implementing website blockers or content filters to restrict access to explicit material.

3. Seeking Professional Help: Consider seeking assistance from a therapist or counselor if efforts to control masturbation are challenging or causing significant distress.

Engaging in cognitive-behavioral therapy to address underlying issues.

4. Self-Compassion: Understand that quitting masturbation can be challenging, and setbacks are common. Approach the process with self-compassion and kindness.

Acknowledging progress and being patient with oneself during the journey.

Quitting masturbation is a personal and sometimes complex endeavor. By identifying triggers, addressing them, and adopting positive habits, individuals can work towards their goals. Seeking professional help and practicing self-compassion are essential components of this journey. Remember that individual experiences may vary, and progress may take time.

Conclusion

Intriguing Masturbation Realities

Here are a few interesting realities to assist you with grasping this issue and its numerous perspectives.

Men who discharge multiple times every week are less inclined to get prostate malignant growth.

Masturbation doesn't bring about penile shrinkage, lessened sex drives, barrenness, or visual deficiency. Ladies in their late twenties stroke off frequently. Masturbation further develops your sexual coexistence. Men jerk off at a higher rate than ladies.

What Causes Masturbation?

Masturbation is extremely regular, and there are a few motivations behind why people make it happen. Here's the reason a great many people make it happen

Discharge strain, absence of sex, worked on comprehension of their bodies, and relationship concerns.

Is there any damage in masturbation?

Indeed, unnecessary masturbation has a few physical and mental unfavorable results.

Actual incidental effects inordinate masturbation can cause edema, culpability sentiments, and skin distress. Oedema is the expanding of body parts brought about by contamination or aggravation. Firmly holding the penis could incite serious enlarging. It could cause skin bothering and tears.

It can likewise cause extraordinary sensations of responsibility, making the individual discouraged or negative about themselves. This can prompt depression and fears, as well as an adjustment of how the person acts in the public eye.

Mental incidental effects unnecessary masturbation is what could be compared to a conflict within. You will see conduct changes like delayed strict convictions, poor sexual correspondence, unnecessary sexual battles with your companion, and relationship inconveniences when your viewpoint of specific things changes.

The most effective method to dispose of Masturbation

On the off chance that masturbation becomes challenging to make due, you have an issue, and here is a simple method for assisting you with controlling it. It might not be an easy task at first, but it is task worth pursuing with patience, determination and faith.

Falling into masturbation while on fight to stop it is totally understandable. It is not a reason to stop the fight. Here are some of the tips that can help in fight against masturbation.

Say no to porn.

Porn is a psychological inspiration for individuals who jerk off often. This mentally affects an individual, impacting how they think and act in the public eye all in all. Keep away from sexual pictures, movies, and sites that could lead you back to that perspective.

Try Something else

One thing that will help you is to redirect your consideration and accomplish something else. Consider taking up another side interest to assist you with supplanting the time you spend jerking off. Start zeroing in on your goals and keep an individual journal.

Letting oneself know that you will succeed makes a big difference for you. This will permit you to zero in your energy on different things as opposed to on masturbation.

Seek expert guidance.

You really want to discuss your concern. You should likewise perceive that you can't fight it single-handedly. A medical care proficient will give you a bunch of directions to help you in managing what is happening.

This can intellectually affect you and leave you with fanatical enthusiastic problem (OCD), which can exacerbate the situation. Make a meeting with a clinician or specialist.

Spend a ton of time mingling.

Did you had any idea that most people try not to mingle in light of the fact that they are forlorn? Indeed, amazing reasoning might really hurt definitely more than you could envision. Mingling permits you to keep your consideration drew in and diverted. So, make it a highlight associate with loved ones or go to the rec center to keep your body dynamic.

Regular actual work

Ordinary activity could assist you with keeping up with your psychological strength. Basic exercises like running, swimming, strolling, and running will support your temperament and assist you with keeping on track. It diminishes strain and keeps your brain clear. Basic exercises for 30 minutes daily will help you.

Inordinate masturbation is a side effect of a fundamental psychological sickness that could prompt social issues. One side effect that masturbation is a habit is areas of strength for an of responsibility following masturbation. This can bring about expanded liquor utilization.

Masturbation turns into an issue in the event that it becomes fanatical or on the other hand assuming you compel yourself to make it happen. It is satisfactory to do as such, yet don't allow it to surpass you.

Note See a specialist before this infection consumes you. Recall that doing so is sound and helpful to everybody, except doing it unnecessarily could prompt further issues.

POEM

Health Benefit of Masturbation

Masturbation, oh masturbation, a topic sometimes met with hesitation,

But let us not forget the benefits, for our health, it truly uplifts.

It can reduce stress and ease the mind, helping us leave our worries behind.

It can improve our sleep at night, and even boost our immune might.

For those with cramps, it can alleviate pain, and may help prevent infections again.

It can also aid in prostate health, and bring pleasure and joy to oneself.

So, don't be shy, give it a try, masturbation can be quite spry,

For health benefits, it's worth a shot, and can even bring pleasure a lot.

Masturbation, oh what a joy, it's more than just a carnal ploy

There are benefits for your health, that can bring you lots of wealth

It helps to relieve stress and tension, and can give you a sense of satisfaction.

It's a natural way to explore, your sexuality and so much more.

Masturbation can improve sleep, and give your immune system a sweep

It's a great way to release hormones, and can even help with headaches and groans

For women, it can help prevent, infections, and keep the area content

For men, it can reduce the risk, of prostate cancer, and give a blissful frisk

So, don't be ashamed or shy, masturbation is healthy, so give it a try

Enjoy the benefits it can provide, and revel in the pleasure it can provide.

Health Challenge of Excessive Masturbation

Masturbation can bring pleasure, it's true, but too much of it can cause issues anew.

It's important to keep things in moderation, and avoid excessive self-gratification.

For some, the health effects can be severe, a challenge that many may sadly fear.

From fatigue to soreness, and even pain, excess masturbation can bring about a strain.

Men may experience problems with their prostate, while women may find themselves in a similar state.

It's important to be aware of these risks, and take steps to avoid any unwanted fixes.

So, remember, while self-love can be great, it's important to not overindulge and tempt fate.

Take care of your body and your health, and enjoy masturbation in moderation, with wealth.

Why to Stop Excessive Masturbation

Masturbation is a natural pleasure, but too much of it can be a measure,

Of problems that can start to appear, if you don't control the urge, my dear.

It's easy to get caught in the act, but don't let it become a daily pact,

For overindulgence can lead to pain, and put your body under strain.

Your mind may wander and lose focus, as you become obsessed with the locus,

Of your desires and urges to fulfill, but too much can lead to a downhill spill.

Your body may weaken and lose its might, as the act of pleasure becomes your sight,

You may feel drained and tired all day, and find it hard to keep the fatigue at bay.

So, take a break, step back, and reflect, on the reasons why you should protect,

Yourself from the dangers of excess, and find balance in your own progress.

Masturbation is healthy when done in moderation, so keep it in check, and avoid frustration,

For a balanced life is what you seek, and your wellbeing is what you must keep.